Costs of Intimate Partner Violence
Against Women in the United States

Department of Health and Human Services
Centers for Disease Control and Prevention
National Center for Injury Prevention and Control

Atlanta, Georgia

March 2003

Costs of Intimate Partner Violence Against Women in the United States is a publication of the National Center for Injury Prevention and Control, part of the Centers for Disease Control and Prevention.

Centers for Disease Control and Prevention
Julie L. Gerberding, MD, MPH
Director

National Center for Injury Prevention and Control
Sue Binder, MD
Director

Division of Violence Prevention
W. Rodney Hammond, PhD
Director

Etiology and Surveillance Branch
Ileana Arias, PhD
Chief

Suggested Citation: National Center for Injury Prevention and Control. *Costs of Intimate Partner Violence Against Women in the United States*. Atlanta (GA): Centers for Disease Control and Prevention; 2003.

Contributors

The following individuals contributed to analyses and research efforts that made this report possible:

Ileana Arias, PhD
National Center for Injury Prevention and Control, CDC

Robert Bardwell, PhD
Bardwell Consulting, Ltd.

Eric Finkelstein, PhD
Research Triangle Institute International

Jacqueline Golding, PhD
University of California, San Francisco

Steven Leadbetter, MS
National Center for Injury Prevention and Control, CDC

Wendy Max, PhD
University of California, San Francisco

Howard Pinderhughes, PhD
University of California, San Francisco

Dorothy Rice, ScD (Hon.)
University of California, San Francisco

Linda E. Saltzman, PhD
National Center for Injury Prevention and Control, CDC

Kevin Tate
Research Triangle Institute International

Nancy Thoennes, PhD
Center for Policy Research

Patricia Tjaden, PhD
Center for Policy Research

Intimate Partner Violence

Acknowledgments

We acknowledge and appreciate the contributions of several CDC colleagues: Sujata Desai, PhD, and Martie Thompson, PhD, for assistance with revisions; Joyce McCurdy, MSA, Melinda Williams, and Chester Pogostin, DVM, MPA, for their coordination efforts; James Mercy, PhD, for scientific review; Marcie-jo Kresnow, MS, for statistical guidance; Lynda Doll, PhD, for facilitating the external review; Phaedra Corso, PhD, for economic consultation; Carole Craft for editing; Alida Knuth and Sandra Emrich for layout and design; and Mary Ann Braun for cover design.

In addition, we extend sincere thanks to Sandra N. Howard, Office of the Assistant Secretary for Planning and Evaluation, Department of Health and Human Services, for her valuable comments and oversight; and to Lois Mock, MA, National Institute of Justice, for coordination efforts.

And we gratefully acknowledge our external peer reviewers:

Elaine Alpert, MD, MPH
Boston University School of Public Health

Jens Ludwig, PhD
Georgetown Public Policy Institute

Anne Menard
Domestic Violence Resource Center

Brian Wiersema
University of Maryland at College Park

Contents

Figures

Intimate Partner Violence

Tables

Costs of Intimate Partner Violence Against Women in the United States: Executive Summary

Background

Although most people believe intimate partner violence (IPV) is a substantial public health problem in the United States, few agree on its magnitude. Recognizing the need to better measure both the scope of the problem of IPV as well as resulting economic costs—in particular, those related to health care—Congress funded the Centers for Disease Control and Prevention (CDC) to conduct a study to obtain national estimates of the occurrence of IPV-related injuries, to estimate their costs to the health care system, and to recommend strategies to prevent IPV and its consequences.

This report—

- Describes briefly the development of the requested study;

- Presents findings for the estimated incidence, prevalence, and costs of nonfatal and fatal IPV;

- Identifies future research needs;

- Highlights CDC's research priorities for IPV prevention.

Incidence, Prevalence, and Consequences of Intimate Partner Violence Against Women in the United States

Data about nonfatal IPV victimizations and resulting health care service use were collected through the National Violence Against Women Survey (NVAWS), funded by the National Institute of Justice and CDC. Based on NVAWS data, an estimated 5.3 million IPV victimizations occur among U.S. women ages 18 and older each year. This violence results in nearly 2.0 million injuries, more than 550,000 of which require medical attention. In addition, IPV victims also lose a total of nearly 8.0 million days of paid work—the equivalent of more than 32,000 full-time jobs—and nearly 5.6 million days of household productivity as a result of the violence.

Data about IPV homicides were obtained from the Federal Bureau of Investigation's Uniform Crime Reports Supplementary Homicide Reports. According to this source, 1,252 women ages 18 and older were killed by an intimate partner in 1995, the same year as incidence data reported in the NVAWS.

Intimate Partner Violence

Costs of Intimate Partner Violence in the United States

The costs of intimate partner rape, physical assault, and stalking exceed $5.8 billion each year, nearly $4.1 billion of which is for direct medical and mental health care services. The total costs of IPV also include nearly $0.9 billion in lost productivity from paid work and household chores for victims of nonfatal IPV and $0.9 billion in lifetime earnings lost by victims of IPV homicide. The largest proportion of the costs is derived from physical assault victimization because that type of IPV is the most prevalent. The largest component of IPV-related costs is health care, which accounts for more than two-thirds of the total costs.

Discussion

Due to exclusions of several cost components about which data were unavailable or insufficient (e.g., certain medical services, social services, criminal justice services), the costs presented in this report likely underestimate the problem of IPV in the U.S. Additionally, because of these omissions, the cost figures here are not comprehensive and should not be used for benefit-cost ratios in analyses of interventions to prevent IPV. However, they can be used to calculate the economic cost savings from reducing IPV and associated injuries, to demonstrate the economic magnitude of IPV, and to evaluate the impact of IPV on a specific sub-sector of the economy, such as consumption of medical resources.

More qualitative and quantitative data are needed to better determine the full magnitude of IPV and associated human and economic costs. There is also a need for primary prevention—preventing IPV from occurring in the first place—rather than focusing only on treating victims and rehabilitating perpetrators after abuse has occurred.

CDC, in its *Injury Research Agenda*, has identified several key areas of research for IPV prevention. These areas include learning how to change social norms that accept intimate partner violence; developing programs for perpetrators and potential perpetrators; increasing our understanding of how violent behaviors toward intimate partners develop; improving collection of data about IPV and its health effects; developing and evaluating training programs for health professionals; and disseminating strategies that work to prevent IPV.

Significant resources for research are needed to better understand the causes and risk factors for IPV and to develop and disseminate effective primary prevention strategies. Until we reduce the incidence of IPV in the United States, we will not reduce the economic and social burden of this problem.

Introduction

Violence against women is a substantial public health problem in the United States. According to data from the criminal justice system, hospital and medical records, mental health records, social services, and surveys, thousands of women are injured or killed each year as a result of violence, many by someone they are involved with or were involved with intimately. Nearly one-third of female homicide victims reported in police records are killed by an intimate partner (Federal Bureau of Investigation 2001).

Intimate partner violence—or IPV—is violence committed by a spouse, ex-spouse, or current or former boyfriend or girlfriend. It occurs among both heterosexual and same-sex couples and is often a repeated offense. Both men and women are victims of IPV, but the literature indicates that women are much more likely than men to suffer physical, and probably psychological, injuries from IPV (Brush 1990; Gelles 1997; Rand and Strom 1997; Rennison and Welchans 2000).

Intimate Partner Violence

Intimate partner violence—also called domestic violence, battering, or spouse abuse—is violence committed by a spouse, ex-spouse, or current or former boyfriend or girlfriend. It can occur among heterosexual or same-sex couples.

IPV results in physical injury, psychological trauma, and sometimes death (Gelles 1997; Kernic, Wolf and Holt 2000; Rennison and Welchans 2000; Sorenson and Saftlas 1994). The consequences of IPV can last a lifetime. Abused women experience more physical health problems and have a higher occurrence of depression, drug and alcohol abuse, and suicide attempts than do women who are not abused (Golding 1996; Campbell, Sullivan and Davidson 1995; Kessler et al. 1994; Kaslow et al. 1998; Moscicki 1989). They also use health care services more often (Miller, Cohen and Rossman 1993).

A growing body of evidence demonstrates the health consequences of intimate partner violence against women (Coker, Smith, Bethea, King and McKeown 2000; Kernic, Wolf and Holt 2000). However, the economic costs of IPV remain largely unknown. Previous cost estimates range from $1.7 billion to $10 billion annually (Straus 1986; Gelles and Straus 1990; Meyer 1992), but they are believed to underestimate the true economic impact of this type of violence (Institute for Women's Policy Research 1995). Researchers have recommended developing national cost estimates for IPV-related medical care, mental health care, police services, social services, and legal services (Gelles and Straus 1990; Straus 1986; Straus and Gelles 1987). However, a recent

Intimate Partner Violence

literature review (Finlayson, Saltzman, Sheridan and Taylor 1999) found only one U.S. study that derived national cost estimates for violence among intimate partners (Miller, Cohen and Wiersema 1996).

Recognizing the need to better measure the magnitude of IPV and resulting economic costs—in particular, those related to health care—the U.S. Congress funded the Centers for Disease Control and Prevention (CDC) to conduct a study to obtain national estimates of the incidence of injuries resulting from IPV, to estimate the costs of injuries to health care facilities, and to recommend strategies to reduce IPV-related injuries and associated costs. Language related to this funding was included in the Violence Against Women Act provisions of the Violent Crime Control and Law Enforcement Act of 1994 (P.L. 103–322).

Given the greater number of IPV-related injuries that occur among women and the instability of cost estimates based on the small numbers of IPV-related injuries among men, this report focuses only on the costs of IPV against women ages 18 and older. Although Congress called only for costs of IPV-related injuries, it was important to include the costs of lost productivity resulting from IPV and to determine the economic costs of lives lost to IPV homicide. These costs contribute significantly to the economic burden of IPV.

This report describes the development of the requested study; presents findings for the estimated incidence, prevalence, and costs of IPV among U.S. adult women; identifies future research needs; and highlights some of CDC's activities related to IPV prevention.

The Need to Estimate the Costs of Intimate Partner Violence

Cost estimates can serve important purposes. For example, they help demonstrate the impact a problem has on society and can shape the attitudes of people who develop public policy and allocate limited funds (Miller, Cohen and Wiersema 1996; Phillips 1987; Snively 1994). They can also help assess the benefit or effectiveness of violence intervention strategies or programs (Haddix, Teutsch, Shaffer and Dunet 1996; Teutsch 1992), which may, in turn, lead to resource allocation to specific programs (Mercy and O'Carroll 1988).

The Need for National Estimates of Intimate Partner Violence

To estimate the costs of IPV, one must first estimate its incidence. While most people acknowledge IPV as a substantial public health problem, few seem to agree on its magnitude (Crowell and Burgess 1996). Several surveys (e.g., Bachman and Saltzman 1995; Rennison and Welchans 2000; Straus and Gelles 1990) have attempted to determine the extent of violence against women, but methods and findings vary considerably, arousing some debate. Many people contend that the magnitude of violence against women—including violence by intimate partners—is underestimated, while others believe it is exaggerated.

Why has the scope of intimate partner violence been so difficult to measure?

Lack of consensus about terminology. Researchers have been unable to agree on a definition of intimate partner violence. In some studies, IPV includes only acts that may cause pain or injury, while ignoring behaviors designed to control or intimidate, such as stalking, humiliation, verbal abuse, imprisonment, and denial of access to money, shelter, or services.

Much of the debate about the number of women affected by intimate partner violence results from this lack of consensus. For example, a researcher who defines IPV more broadly—including stalking and other forms of psychological abuse, as well as physical and sexual violence—will produce a larger estimate than a researcher who uses a more narrow definition that includes physical and sexual violence only (DeKeseredy 2000). A definition that separately measures component types of violence—physical, sexual, and emotional—will also likely produce different measurements than one that combines all types of violence (Gordon 2000).

Variations in survey methodology. Sampling strategies and how the purpose of a survey is explained may affect how participants answer survey questions. For example, a respondent on the National Crime Victimization Survey may not acknowledge being the victim of IPV if he or she does not believe IPV is a crime. However, the same respondent might disclose IPV victimization on a survey about family conflict.

Gaps in data collection. Because no national system exists for ongoing collection of data about IPV against women, estimates are often drawn from data gathered for other purposes. For example, hospitals collect information about victims to provide patient care and for billing purposes; they may record few details about the violence itself or about the perpetrator and his or her relationship to the victim. In contrast, police collect data that will aid in apprehending the perpetrator, and thus may collect little information about the victim.

Different time frames. Studies of IPV have used different time frames to study victimization. Some measure lifetime victimization, while others measure annual victimization. These differences are not always well understood and have sometimes resulted in inappropriate comparisons being drawn between studies that are not in fact comparable.

Reluctance to report victimization. Many victims do not want to report IPV because they may fear, love, depend on, or wish to protect the perpetrator. When medical care is required, women may attribute their injuries to other causes.

Repetitive nature of IPV. Often, IPV involves repetitive behavior, rather than a single incident. However, reports about IPV do not always clearly indicate whether data refer to the number of IPV incidents or the number of victims.

Limited populations. Previous studies have focused either on married or cohabiting couples or on dating relationships. Although a few studies have looked at violence among same-sex couples, most research has examined only heterosexual relationships. Few studies have examined IPV among the population overall.

Survey limitations. Many data about IPV have been collected through surveys, which rely on self-reports by victims. These self-reports may not accurately reflect the magnitude of the problem, if respondents do not answer questions truthfully or do not accurately recall events. Additionally, despite carefully worded questions and efforts to ensure that participants understand what is being asked, respondents may interpret terms differently.

Because methodological differences such as those described here can affect the findings of a survey or study, researchers must explain the choice of a particular methodology, define terms used, and clearly explain how information was gathered (CDC 2000). This information allows others to examine findings in the context in which data were collected and can help readers understand how the findings compare with those of other surveys or studies. In keeping with this practice, this report specifies the methodology employed and the definitions used.

The National Violence Against Women Survey

When Congress requested a study about the costs of IPV, no existing survey or study had a large enough sample to reliably estimate the occurrence of IPV-related injuries in the U.S. population. Nor did any existing survey or study include enough information about the nature and extent of injuries and their treatment to make the national projections Congress had requested. A new study was needed to fill gaps in knowledge about the magnitude of IPV.

Developing and Implementing the National Violence Against Women Survey

CDC learned that the National Institute of Justice (NIJ), the research arm of the U.S. Department of Justice, had funded Patricia Tjaden and Nancy Thoennes of the Center for Policy Research in Denver to develop the National Violence Against Women Survey—or NVAWS. The NVAWS was to generate information about the incidence, prevalence, characteristics, and consequences of physical assault, rape, and stalking perpetrated against U.S. women ages 18 and older by all types of perpetrators, including intimate partners.

Rather than duplicating efforts, CDC approached NIJ about supplementing its grant to Tjaden and Thoennes to broaden the size and scope of the survey by increasing the sample size, conducting a companion survey of male respondents, and adding questions about violence in same-sex intimate relationships. The broader survey could then be used as the basis for calculating more reliable cost estimates of IPV and other forms of violence. Both NIJ and the Center for Policy Research agreed to delay the survey to accommodate a supplemental award and make CDC's proposed changes.

The supplemental funds expanded the survey population to a number large enough to provide reliable national estimates of the incidence and prevalence of forcible rapes, physical assault, and stalking; related injuries and health care costs, including those for mental health care services; and indirect costs due to lost productivity of paid work and household chores.

CDC and the office of the Assistant Secretary for Planning and Evaluation, another component of HHS, contracted with Wendy Max, Dorothy Rice, Jacqueline Golding, and Howard Pinderhughes at the University of California, San Francisco, to use the methodology they had developed earlier (Rice et al. 1996) to review draft survey questions and to recommend changes that would enable cost data to be collected with the NVAWS. The survey questions sought to detail the type of violence; the circumstances surrounding the violence; the relationship between victim and perpetrator; and consequences to the victim, including injuries sustained, use of medical and mental health care services, contact with the criminal justice system, and time lost from usual activities.

From November 1995 to May 1996, a national probability sample of 8,000 women and 8,000 men ages 18 and older were surveyed via telephone using a computer-assisted interviewing system. Female interviewers surveyed female respondents. A Spanish-language version of the survey was used with Spanish-speaking respondents.

In addition to the 8,000 completed interviews, the women's survey contacts included 4,829 ineligible households; 4,608 eligible households that refused to participate; and 351 interviews that were terminated before completion. The women's response rate was 71.0%.

Analyzing NVAWS Data and Estimating the Costs of Intimate Partner Violence

Tjaden and Thoennes (1999) used the NVAWS data and U.S. Census figures for the population of women ages 18 and older to generate national estimates of the incidence and prevalence of IPV-related injuries among women.[1] Cost estimates were to be derived from these estimates. Max and colleagues (1999) applied their previously developed methodology for estimating the costs of intimate partner violence to the NVAWS incidence data and data from other sources (Rice, Max, Golding and Pinderhughes 1996).

---

[1]This report used only the data about violence committed against women by intimate partners. However, NVAWS data have also provided insight into other areas of violence, including a comparison of women's and men's experiences as victims of rape, physical assault, and stalking by all types of perpetrators.

Intimate Partner Violence

CDC funded Research Triangle Institute International (RTI) to derive measures of reliability for the incidence, prevalence, and cost estimates. Additionally, Max and colleagues and RTI developed estimates of the present value of lifetime earnings for fatal IPV by combining economic data with IPV homicide data from the Federal Bureau of Investigation.

The report that follows reflects CDC's integration of the work by Tjaden and Thoennes, Max and colleagues, and RTI.

Definitions Used in the NVAWS and this Report

Throughout this report, one will read about intimate partner violence (IPV) and specific types of violent behaviors, as well as about incidence, prevalence, and victimization rates of IPV. As stated earlier, there is a lack of consensus about IPV-related terminology. Therefore, it is important to define those terms as they were used in the NVAWS to ensure that readers have a consistent understanding of what they mean and to allow readers to compare findings presented in this report with those of other studies.

Intimate partner violence (IPV) against women includes rape, physical assault, and stalking perpetrated by a current or former date, boyfriend, husband, or cohabiting partner, with cohabiting meaning living together as a couple. Both same-sex and opposite-sex cohabitants are included in the definition. This definition of IPV resembles the one developed by CDC (Saltzman et al. 1999); however, it also includes stalking because of the high level of fear that stalking generally provokes in women and the associated costs that may result.

Rape is the use of force, without the victim's consent, or threat of force to penetrate the victim's vagina or anus by penis, tongue, fingers, or object, or the victim's mouth by penis. The definition includes both attempted and completed acts. This definition is similar to that used in the National Women's Study (National Victim Center and Crime Victims Research and Treatment Center 1992) and is roughly equivalent to what the justice system refers to as rape or attempted rape.

Physical assault is any behavior that inflicts physical harm or threatens or attempts to do so. Specific behaviors include throwing something at the victim; pushing, grabbing, or shoving; pulling hair; slapping, hitting, kicking, or biting; choking or trying to drown; hitting with an object; beating up the victim; threatening with a gun or knife; and shooting or stabbing the victim. This definition is similar to that used in the National Family Violence Survey (Straus and Gelles 1986) and the Canadian Violence Against Women Survey (Johnson 1996), and it is roughly equivalent to what the justice system refers to as simple and aggravated assault.

Stalking is repeated visual or physical proximity, non-consensual communication, and/or verbal, written, or implied threats directed at a specific individual that would arouse fear in a reasonable person. The stalker need not make a credible threat of violence against the victim, but the victim must experience a high level of fear or feel that they or someone close to them will be harmed or killed by the stalker. This definition is similar to that used in the model anti-stalking legislation developed for states by NIJ (National Criminal Justice Association 1993).

Prevalence is the number of U.S. women ages 18 and older who have been victimized by an intimate partner at some point during their lifetimes (lifetime prevalence) or during the 12 months preceding the NVAWS (past 12 months prevalence). In this report, prevalence refers to past 12 months prevalence unless otherwise specified.

Incidence is the number of separate episodes of IPV that occurred among U.S. women ages 18 and older during the 12 months preceding the survey. For IPV, incidence frequently exceeds prevalence because IPV is often repeated. In other words, one victim (who is counted once under the prevalence definition) may experience several victimizations over the course of 12 months (each of which contributes to the incidence count).

Victimization rate is the number of IPV victimizations involving U.S. women ages 18 and older per 1,000 women in that population. The population estimate used in this report is the U.S. Census Bureau's projection of 100,697,000 women ages 18 and older in 1995.

A Note About Annual Estimates

This report presents annual data about IPV and its costs, generalized from data about the incidence of intimate partner violence in a given year (1995) and the costs associated with those victimizations. CDC acknowledges that the health care costs, value of lost productivity, and present value of lifetime earnings among IPV murder victims may be different today than in 1995. However, this report reflects the most appropriate, reliable data currently available about the costs associated with IPV.

Intimate Partner Violence

References

Bachman R, Saltzman L. *Violence Against Women: Estimates From the Redesigned Survey*. U.S. Department of Justice, Bureau of Justice Statistics, NCJ 154348; 1995.

Brush LD. Violent acts and injurious outcomes in married couples: methodological issues in the National Survey of Families and Households. *Gender and Society* 1990;4(1):56–67.

Campbell J, Sullivan CM, Davidson WD. Women who use domestic violence shelters: changes in depression over time. *Psychology of Women Quarterly* 1995;19:237–55.

Centers for Disease Control and Prevention. Building data systems for monitoring and responding to violence against women: recommendations from a workshop. *Morbidity and Mortality Weekly Report* 2000;49(RR-11):1–16.

Coker AL, Smith PH, Bethea L, King MR, McKeown RE. Physical health consequences of physical and psychological intimate partner violence. *Archives of Family Medicine* 2000;9:451–7.

Crowell N, Burgess A, editors; National Research Council. *Understanding Violence Against Women*. Washington (DC): National Academy Press; 1996.

DeKeseredy WS. Current controversies on defining nonlethal violence against women in intimate heterosexual relationships: empirical implications. *Violence Against Women* 2000;6(7):728–46.

Federal Bureau of Investigation. Crime in the United States 2000. *Uniform Crime Reports*. Washington (DC): U.S. Department of Justice; 2001.

Finlayson TJ, Saltzman LE, Sheridan DJ, Taylor WK. Estimating hospital charges associated with intimate violence. *Violence Against Women* 1999;5(3):313–35.

Gelles RJ. *Intimate Violence in Families*. 3rd ed. Thousand Oaks (CA): Sage Publications; 1997.

Gelles RJ, Straus MA. The medical and psychological costs of family violence. In: Straus MA, Gelles RJ, editors. *Physical Violence in American Families: Risk Factors in Adaptations to Violence in 8,145 Families*. New Brunswick (NJ): Transaction Publishers; 1990. p. 425–30.

Golding JM. Sexual assault history and limitations in physical functioning in two general population samples. *Research in Nursing and Health* 1996;19:33–44.

Gordon M. Definitional issues in violence against women: surveillance and research from a violence research perspective. *Violence Against Women* 2000;6(7):747–83.

Haddix AC, Teutsch SM, Shaffer PA, Dunet DO. *Prevention Effectiveness: A Guide to Decision Analysis and Economic Evaluation*. New York: Oxford University Press; 1996.

Institute for Women's Policy Research. *Measuring the Costs of Domestic Violence and the Cost-Effectiveness of Interventions: An Initial Assessment of the State of the Art and Proposals for Future Research*. Victim Services, Inc. Unpublished; 1995.

Johnson H. *Dangerous Domains: Violence Against Women in Canada*. Toronto: Nelson Canada; 1996.

Kaslow N, Thompson MP, Meadows L, Jacobs D, Chance S, Gibb B, et al. Factors that mediate or moderate the link between partner abuse and suicidal behavior in African American women. *Journal of Consulting and Clinical Psychology* 1998;66:533–40.

Kernic MA, Wolf ME, Holt VL. Rates and relative risk of hospital admission among women in violent intimate partner relationships. *American Journal of Public Health* 2000;90(9):1416–20.

Kessler RC, McGonagle KA, Zhao S, Nelson CB, Hughes M, Eshleman S, et al. Lifetime and 12-month prevalence of DSM-III-R psychiatric disorders in the United States: results from the National Comorbidity Survey. *Archives of General Psychiatry* 1994;51:8–19.

Max W, Rice D, Golding J, Pinderhughes H. *The Cost of Intimate Partner Violence in the United States, 1995*; 1999. Unpublished report for contract 282-92-0048, funded by the Office of the Assistant Secretary for Planning and Evaluation and the Centers for Disease Control and Prevention, U.S. Department of Health and Human Services.

Mercy JA, O'Carroll P. New directions in violence prediction: the public health arena. *Violence and Victims* 1988;3:285–301.

Meyer H. The billion dollar epidemic. *American Medical News* 1992 January 6.

Miller T, Cohen MA, Rossman SB. Victim costs of violent crime and resulting injuries. *Health Affairs* 1993;12(4):186–97.

Miller TR, Cohen MA, Wiersema B. *Victim Costs and Consequences: A New Look*. National Institute of Justice Research Report. Washington (DC): National Institute of Justice, U.S. Department of Justice; 1996. NCJ 155282.

Moscicki ED. Epidemiologic surveys as tools for studying suicidal behavior: a review. *Suicide and Life-Threatening Behavior* 1989;19:131–46.

National Criminal Justice Association. Project to Develop a Model Anti-stalking Code for States. Washington (DC): U.S. Department of Justice, National Institute of Justice; 1993.

National Victim Center and the Crime Victims Research and Treatment Center. *Rape in America: A Report to the Nation.* Arlington (VA): The Centers; 1992.

Phillips MA. Why do costings? *Health Policy and Planning* 1987;2;255–7.

Rand M, Strom K. *Violence-Related Injuries Treated in Hospital Emergency Departments.* Washington (DC): Bureau of Justice Statistics, U.S. Department of Justice: 1997. NCJ 156921.

Rennison CM, Welchans S. *Intimate Partner Violence.* Washington (DC): Bureau of Justice Statistics, U.S. Department of Justice; 2000. NCJ 178247.

Rice DP, Max W, Golding J, Pinderhughes H. *The Cost of Domestic Violence to the Health Care System;* 1996. Final Report for contract 282-92-0048, funded by the Office of the Assistant Secretary for Planning and Evaluation, in consultation with the Centers for Disease Control and Prevention.

Saltzman LE, Fanslow JL, McMahon PM, Shelley GA. *Intimate Partner Violence Surveillance: Uniform definitions and recommended data elements, Version 1.0.* Atlanta: Centers for Disease Control and Prevention, National Center for Injury Prevention and Control; 1999.

Snively S. *The New Zealand Economic Cost of Family Violence.* Wellington (New Zealand): Family Violence Unit, Department of Social Welfare; 1994.

Straus MA. Medical care costs of intrafamily assault and homicide. *Bulletin of the New York Academy of Medicine* 1986;62(5):556–61.

Straus MA, Gelles RJ. Societal change and change in family violence from 1975 to 1985 as revealed by two national surveys. *Journal of Marriage and the Family* 1986;48:465–79.

Straus MA, Gelles RJ. The costs of family violence. *Public Health Reports* 1987;102: 638–41.

Straus MA, Gelles RJ. How violent are American families? Estimates from the National Family Violence Resurvey and other studies. In: Straus MA, Gelles RJ, editors. *Physical Violence in American Families: Risk Factors and Adaptations to Violence in 8,145 Families.* New Brunswick (NJ): Transaction Publishers; 1990. p. 95–112.

Teutsch SM. A framework for assessing the effectiveness of disease and injury prevention. *Morbidity and Mortality Weekly Report* 1992;41(RR-3);1–13.

Tjaden P, Thoennes N. *Prevalence, Incidence, and Consequences of Intimate Partner Violence Against Women: Findings from the National Violence Against Women Survey;* 1999. Unpublished report for grant 93-IJ-CX-0012, funded by the Centers for Disease Control and Prevention.

Incidence, Prevalence, and Consequences of Intimate Partner Violence Against Women in the United States

Before estimating the costs of intimate partner violence, one needs to know how many women were injured nonfatally as a result of IPV; how many women used medical and mental health care services after IPV victimization; and how many women lost time from paid work and household chores after IPV. The National Violence Against Women Survey (NVAWS) provided that information. One also needs to know how many women died as a result of IPV. This information was obtained from the FBI's Uniform Crime Reports Supplementary Homicide Reports (Fox 2000).

This chapter describes the findings of the NVAWS, along with the national estimates calculated from those findings. It also presents estimates of the number of IPV homicides. The data presented reflect the incidence of IPV and related health care service use in 1995; these data are the most appropriate, reliable data currently available about the health care costs associated with IPV.

Incidence and Prevalence of Nonfatal Intimate Partner Rape, Physical Assault, and Stalking

The NVAWS asked the 8,000 U.S. women ages 18 and older if they had been victims of IPV at any time in their lives or within the 12 months preceding the survey.

Intimate partner rape. Of the female NVAWS respondents, 7.7% had been raped by an intimate partner at some point in their lifetimes; 0.2% reported intimate partner rape in the past 12 months.[1] Extrapolating these percentages to U.S. Census population data, nearly 7.8 million women have been raped by an intimate partner at some time in their lives, and an estimated 201,394 women are raped by an intimate partner each year (Table 1).

Because some respondents reported multiple intimate partner rapes in the 12 months preceding the survey, the incidence of rape exceeded the prevalence. Women who were raped in that year experienced an average of 1.6 victimizations. This calculates to an

---

[1] Only 16 women participating in the NVAWS reported IPV rape in the 12 months preceding the survey. Estimates based on this small number are marginally stable and should be viewed with caution.

estimated 322,230 rapes by intimate partners each year, an annual victimization rate of 3.2 intimate partner rapes per 1,000 women [322,230 rapes / 100,697,000 women = 0.0032 or 3.2 per 1000] (Table 2).

Intimate partner physical assault. The NVAWS found that 22.1% of women had been physically assaulted by an intimate partner at some time in their lives, and 1.3% reported such an event in the 12 months preceding the survey. Thus, an estimated 1.3 million women are victims of physical assault by an intimate partner each year (Table 1).

Women who were physically assaulted by an intimate partner in the previous 12 months experienced an average of 3.4 separate assaults. Using these data, an estimated 4.5 million IPV physical assaults occur annually, a victimization rate of 44.2 per 1,000 (Table 2).

Intimate partner stalking. The survey found that 4.8% of women reported being stalked by an intimate partner at some time in their lives. One-half percent of women had been stalked in the 12 months preceding the survey, which equates to an estimated 503,485 women stalked by intimate partners each year (Table 1).

Because stalking, by definition, involves repeated acts of harassment and intimidation, and because no woman in the NVAWS reported being stalked by more than one intimate partner in the 12 months preceding the survey, the incidence and prevalence of intimate partner stalking are identical. Thus, the annual victimization rate for intimate partner stalking among women is 5.0 per 1,000 (Table 2).

Injuries Among Victims of Intimate Partner Violence

To explore the extent and nature of injuries associated with intimate partner violence, respondents disclosing rape or physical assault were asked whether they were injured during their most recent victimization, and if so, what types of injuries they sustained. Victims of stalking were not asked about injuries because the NVAWS definition of stalking does not include behaviors that inflict physical harm.

The NVAWS found that 36.2% of the women who were raped by an intimate partner sustained an injury (other than the rape itself) during their most recent victimization (Figure 1), and 41.5% of physical assault victims were injured (Figure 2). The majority of women who were injured during the most recent IPV episode sustained relatively minor injuries, such as scratches, bruises, and welts. Relatively few women sustained more serious types of injuries, such as lacerations, broken bones, dislocated joints, head or spinal cord injuries, chipped or broken teeth, or internal injuries.[2]

---

[2]For information about specific injuries, see Tjaden P, Thoennes N. *Extent, Nature, and Consequences of Intimate Partner Violence: Findings from the National Violence Against Women Survey.* Washington (DC): U.S. Department of Justice, Office of Justice Programs, National Institute of Justice; 2000. NCJ 181867.

Victims' Use of
Medical Care Services

Respondents who were injured were asked if they received medical treatment and, if so, what type of care.[3]

NVAWS Findings

Of the women injured during their most recent intimate partner rape, 31.0% received some type of medical care, such as ambulance/paramedic services, treatment in a hospital emergency department (ED), or physical therapy (Figure 1). A comparable proportion (28.1%) of IPV physical assault victims who were injured received some type of medical care (Figure 2).

More than three-quarters of the rape and physical assault victims who received medical care were treated in a hospital setting (79.6% and 78.6%, respectively). Among women seeking medical care, 51.3% of rape victims and 59.1% of physical assault victims were treated in an ED, while 30.8% of rape victims and 24.2% of physical assault victims received some other type of outpatient service. Of those who were treated in a hospital, 43.6% of rape and 32.6% of physical assault victims were admitted and spent one or more nights in the hospital (Figures 1 and 2).

National Estimates of
Medical Care Service Use

Of the estimated 322,230 intimate partner rapes each year, 116,647 result in injuries (other than the rape itself), 36,161 of which require medical care. And of the nearly 4.5 million physical assault victimizations, more than 1.8 million cause injuries, 519,031 of which require medical care. Nearly 15,000 rape victimizations and more than 240,000 physical assault victimizations result in hospital ED visits (Table 3).

Multiple medical care visits are often required for each IPV victimization. For example, victims of both rape and physical assault averaged 1.9 hospital ED visits per victimization, resulting in an estimated 486,151 visits each year to hospital EDs resulting from rape and physical assault victimizations (Table 4). Consequently, the total number of medical service uses exceeds the total number of victimizations resulting in medical care.

---

[3]To yield more reliable estimates for service use, all most-recent IPV victimizations reported in the NVAWS—including those that occurred more than 12 months before the interview—were used to establish use patterns.

Figure 1.
Percentage Distributions of U.S. Adult Female Victims of
Intimate Partner Rape by Medical Care Service Use, 1995

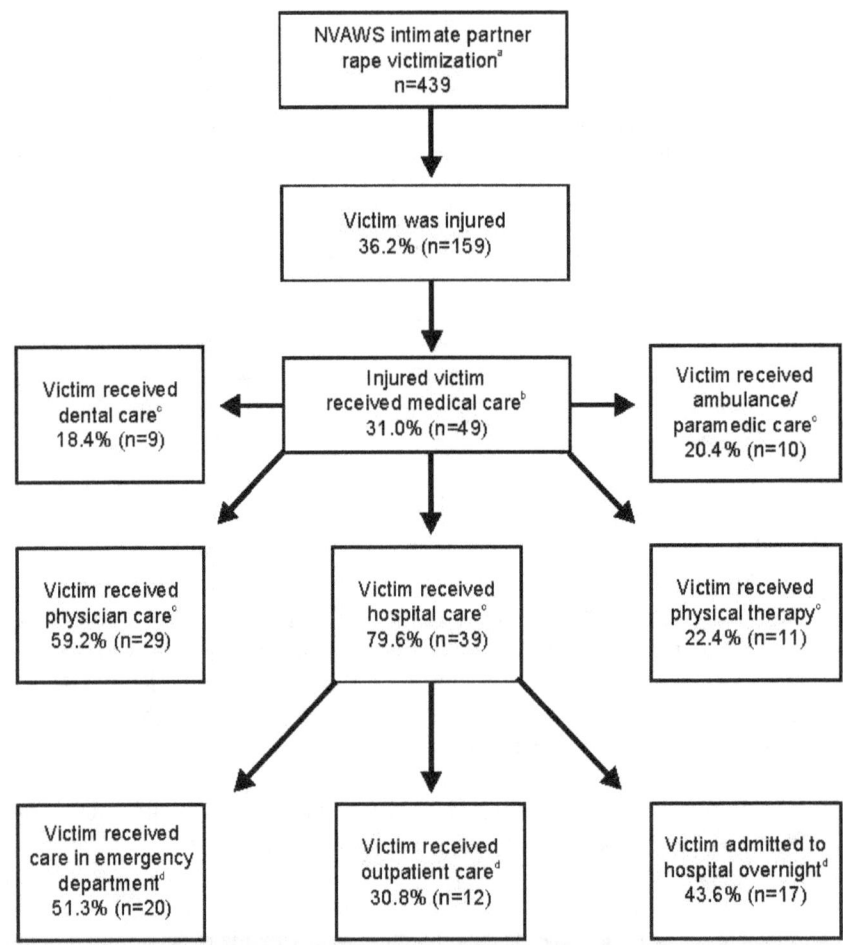

[a] Estimates are based on the most recent intimate partner victimization since the age of 18.
[b] The percentage of victims who received medical care is based on 158 responses from victims who were injured, excluding one "don't know" response.
[c] Estimates are based on responses from victims who received medical care.
[d] Estimates are based on responses from victims who received hospital care.

Note: Total percentages for type of medical and hospital care received exceed 100 because some victims had multiple forms of medical/hospital care.

Sources: Tjaden and Thoennes 2000; Bardwell Consulting, Ltd. (unpublished data) 2001.

Figure 2.
Percentage Distributions of U.S. Adult Female Victims of
Intimate Partner Physical Assault by Medical Care Service Use, 1995

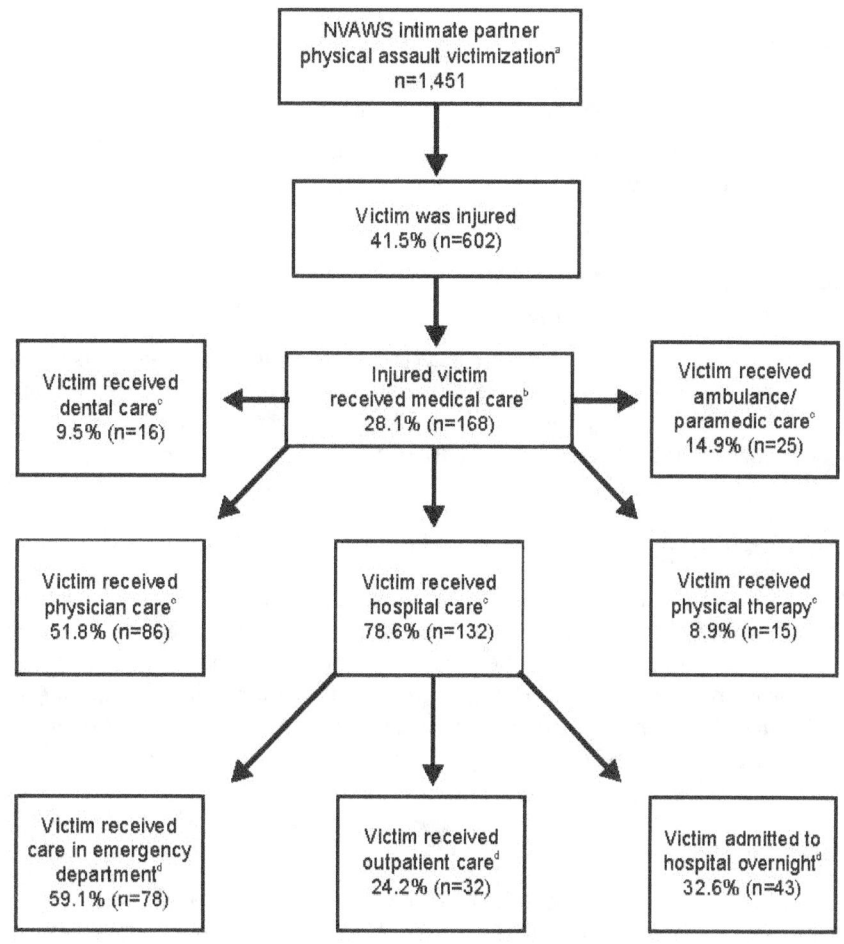

[a]Estimates are based on the most recent intimate partner victimization since the age of 18.
[b] The percentage of victims who received medical care is based on 598 responses from victims who were injured, excluding 4 "don't know" responses.
[c]Estimates are based on 168 responses from victims who received medical care, although the percentage of victims who received physician care is based on 166 respondents, excluding 2 "don't know" responses.
[d] Estimates are based on responses from victims who received hospital care.

Note: Total percentages for type of medical and hospital care received exceed 100 because some victims had multiple forms of medical/hospital care.

Sources: Tjaden and Thoennes 2000; Bardwell Consulting, Ltd. (unpublished data) 2001.

Intimate Partner Violence

Victims' Use of Mental Health Care Services

NVAWS respondents who were victimized by an intimate partner were asked whether they talked to a psychologist, psychiatrist, or other type of mental health professional about their most recent victimization, and if so, how many times.

NVAWS Findings

One-third of female rape victims, 26.4% of physical assault victims, and 42.6% of stalking victims said they talked to a mental health professional, most of them multiple times. Among these women, rape victims averaged 12.4 visits, physical assault victims averaged 12.9 visits, and stalking victims averaged 9.6 visits (Table 5).

National Estimates of Mental Health Care Service Use

Of the estimated 5.3 million rapes, physical assaults, or stalking incidents by intimate partners each year, nearly 1.5 million result in some type of mental health counseling. The total number of mental health care visits by female IPV victims each year is estimated to be more than 18.5 million (Table 5).

Victims' Lost Productivity

The NVAWS asked IPV victims whether their most recent victimization caused them to lose time from routine activities, including employment, household chores, and childcare. Victims who lost time from employment and household chores were asked how many days they lost from these activities. This information was then applied to the estimated number of women victimized each year by intimate partners to produce annual estimates of total lost productivity.

NVAWS Findings

Of adult female IPV victims, 35.3% who were stalked, 21.5% who were raped, and 17.5% who were physically assaulted lost time from paid work (Table 6). Women stalked by an intimate partner averaged the largest number of days lost from paid work (10.1). Women raped by an intimate partner lost an average 8.1 days from paid work, and victims of IPV physical assault lost 7.2 days on average per victimization (Table 7).

Among IPV stalking victims, 17.5% lost days from household chores; IPV rape and physical assault victims lost 13.5% and 10.3% respectively (Table 6). Victims of IPV rape lost the largest average number of days from household chores (13.5), followed by stalking (12.7) and physical assault (8.4) victims (Table 7).

National Estimates of Lost Productivity

According to NVAWS estimates, U.S. women lose nearly 8.0 million days of paid work each year because of violence perpetrated against them by current or former husbands, cohabitants, dates, and boyfriends. This is the equivalent of 32,114 full-time jobs each year. An additional 5.6 million days are lost from household chores (Table 7).

Intimate Partner Homicides Among Women

Data about fatal IPV were obtained from the Federal Bureau of Investigation's Uniform Crime Reports (UCR) Supplementary Homicide Reports. Data in the UCR are submitted to the FBI by nearly 17,000 law enforcement agencies nationwide. In 1995, the same year as data from the NVAWS, 1,252 U.S. women ages 18 and older were killed by intimate partners.

Summary

Nearly 5.3 million intimate partner victimizations occur among U.S. women ages 18 and older each year. This violence results in nearly 2.0 million injuries and nearly 1,300 deaths. Of the IPV injuries, more than 555,000 require medical attention, and more than 145,000 are serious enough to warrant hospitalization for one or more nights. IPV also results in more than 18.5 million mental health care visits each year. Add to that the 13.6 million days of lost productivity from paid work and household chores among IPV survivors and the value of IPV murder victims' expected lifetime earnings, and it is clear to see that intimate partner violence against women places a significant burden on society.

References

Bardwell Consulting, Ltd. Unpublished data for task order 0621-15, funded by the Centers for Disease Control and Prevention; 2001.

Fox JA. Uniform Crime Reports [United States]: Supplementary Homicide Reports, 1976–1998 [Computer file]. ICPSR version. Boston (MA): Northeastern University, College of Criminal Justice [producer]. 2000. Ann Arbor (MI): Inter-University Consortium for Political and Social Research [distributor]. 2000. Available from: URL: http://www.icpsr.umich.edu:8080/ICPSR-STUDY/03000.xml.

Intimate Partner Violence

Max W, Rice DP, Golding J, Pinderhughes H. *Cost of Intimate Partner Violence Against Women in the United States, 1995*; 1999. Unpublished report for contract 282-92-0048, funded by the Office of the Assistant Secretary for Planning and Evaluation and the Centers for Disease Control and Prevention, U.S. Department of Health and Human Services.

Tjaden P, Thoennes N. *Prevalence, Incidence, and Consequences of Intimate Partner Violence Against Women: Findings from the National Violence Against Women Survey*; 1999. Unpublished report for grant 93-IJ-CX-0012, funded by the U.S. Department of Justice, National Institute of Justice; and the Centers for Disease Control and Prevention.

Tjaden P, Thoennes N. *Extent, Nature, and Consequences of Intimate Partner Violence*: *Findings from the National Violence Against Women Survey*. Washington (DC): U.S. Department of Justice, Office of Justice Programs, National Institute of Justice; 2000. NCJ 181867.

Wetrogen SI. *Projections of the Population of States by Age, Sex, and Race: 1988 to 2010*, Current Population Reports, P25-1017. Washington (DC): U.S. Bureau of the Census; 1988.

Table 1. Percentage of NVAWS Respondents and Estimated Number of U.S. Adult Women Nonfatally Victimized by an Intimate Partner in Their Lifetimes and in the Previous 12 Months, by Type of Victimization, 1995

Type of Victimization	In Lifetime		In Previous 12 Months	
	Percent in NVAWS[a]	Estimated No. Women[b]	Percent in NVAWS[a]	Estimated No. Women[b]
Rape	7.7	7,753,669	0.2[c]	201,394
Physical assault	22.1	22,254,037	1.3	1,309,061
Stalking	4.8	4,833,456	0.5	503,485
TOTAL Victimized[d]	**25.5**	**25,677,735**	**1.8**	**1,812,546**

[a]Percentage of respondents is based on NVAWS interviews with 8,000 U.S. women ages 18 and older.

[b]Estimated number of women is calculated by applying the NVAWS percentage to the 1995 projected population estimate of women ages 18 and older in the U.S. (100,697,000).

[c]Only 16 women participating in the NVAWS reported IPV rape in the 12 months preceding the survey. Estimates based on this small number are marginally stable and should be viewed with caution.

[d]The individual types of victimizations do not sum to the total number of women victimized because some victims reported multiple types of victimization.

Sources: Tjaden and Thoennes 2000; Wetrogen 1988.

Table 2. Estimated Number of Nonfatal Intimate Partner Rape, Physical Assault, and Stalking Victimizations Against U.S. Adult Women, 1995

Type of Victimization	No. of Victims	Average No. of Victimizations Per Victim[a]	Total No. of Victimizations	Annual Rate of Victimization Per 1,000 Women
Rape	201,394	1.6	322,230[b]	3.2[b]
Physical assault	1,309,061	3.4	4,450,807	44.2
Stalking	503,485	1.0	503,485	5.0

[a]The average number of victimizations per victim is based on the previous 12 months. Because stalking by definition means repeated acts, and because no woman was stalked by more than one intimate partner in the 12 months preceding the survey, the number of stalking victimizations was imputed to be the same as the number of stalking victims. Thus, the average number of stalking victimizations per victim is 1.0.

[b]Relative standard error exceeds 30 percent. Based on 16 women who reported intimate partner rape in the previous 12 months, this estimate is unstable and used only as part of intermediate calculations to determine the total costs associated with IPV.

Sources: Tjaden and Thoennes 2000; Bardwell Consulting, Ltd. (unpublished data) 2001.

Table 3. Estimated Victimization Outcomes and Medical Care Service Use by U.S. Adult Female Victims of Nonfatal Intimate Partner Rape and Physical Assault, 1995

Victimization Outcomes and Medical Services Used	Rape	Physical Assault	Total
Victimizations	322,230	4,450,807	4,773,037
Victimization resulting in injury[a]	116,647	1,847,085	1,963,732
Victimization resulting in some type of medical care[b]	36,161	519,031	555,192
Victimization resulting in:			
Hospital care[c]	28,784	407,958	436,742
Physician care[c]	21,407	268,858	290,265
Dental care[c]	6,654	49,308	55,962
Ambulance/paramedic care[c]	7,377	77,336	84,713
Physical therapy[c]	8,100	46,194	54,294
Victimization resulting in hospital:			
ED care[d]	14,766	241,103	255,869
Outpatient care[d]	8,865	98,726	107,591
Overnight care[d]	12,550	132,994	145,544

[a]Derived by applying the injury percentages (Figures 1 and 2) to the total number of victimizations.

[b]Derived by applying the medical care percentages (Figures 1 and 2) to the number of victimizations resulting in injury.

[c]The number of victimizations resulting in each particular type of medical care (e.g., physician care) was derived by applying the percentage of victimizations resulting in that particular service (Figures 1 and 2) to the overall number of victimizations resulting in some type of medical care.

[d]The number of victimizations resulting in each particular type of hospital care (e.g., ED care) was derived by applying the percentage of victimizations resulting in that particular type of care (Figures 1 and 2) to the overall number of victimizations resulting in hospital care.

Sources: Tjaden and Thoennes 2000; Bardwell Consulting, Ltd. (unpublished data) 2001; Max, Rice, Golding and Pinderhughes (unpublished data) 1999.

Table 4. Estimated Average and Total Number of Medical Care Service Uses by U.S. Adult Female Victims of Nonfatal Intimate Partner Rape and Physical Assault, 1995

Type of Medical Service	Rape		Physical Assault		Rape and Physical Assault
	Average No. of Uses	Total No. of Uses[a]	Average No. of Uses	Total No. of Uses[a]	Total No. of Uses
ED visits	1.9	28,055	1.9	458,096	486,151
Outpatient visits	1.6	14,184	3.1	306,051	320,235
Hospital overnights	3.9	48,945	5.7	758,066	807,011
Physician visits	5.2	111,316	3.2	860,346	971,662
Dental visits	2.3	15,304	4.4	216,955	232,259
Ambulance/paramedic services	1.3	9,950	1.1	85,070	95,020
Physical therapy visits	13.4	108,540	21.1	974,693	1,083,233

[a]The total number of uses for each type of medical care service for rape and physical assault victimizations was derived by multiplying the total number of victimizations resulting in that medical care service (Table 3) by the average number of uses of that service.

NOTE: Estimates were derived separately for each type of victimization. Overall totals for service use were subsequently derived by summing the respective estimates across victimization types. Consequently, the overall average number of medical care service uses was not derived.

Sources: Tjaden and Thoennes 2000; Bardwell Consulting, Ltd. (unpublished data) 2001; Max, Rice, Golding and Pinderhughes (unpublished data) 1999.

Intimate Partner Violence

Table 5. Estimates of Mental Health Care Service Use by U.S. Adult Female Victims of Intimate Partner Violence by Victimization Type, 1995

Victimization and Mental Health Use Estimates	Rape	Physical Assault	Stalking	Total
Total number of victimizations	322,230	4,450,807	503,485	5,276,522
Percent of victimizations resulting in mental health care services	33.0%	26.4%	42.6%	N/A
Number of victimizations resulting in mental health care services	106,336	1,175,013	214,485	1,495,834
Average number of mental health care visits per victimization	12.4	12.9	9.6	N/A
TOTAL number of mental health care visits	1,318,566	15,157,668	2,059,056	18,535,290

NOTE: Estimates were derived separately for each type of victimization. Overall totals for victimizations and mental health care visits were subsequently derived by summing the respective estimates across victimization types. Consequently, the overall percentage receiving mental health care services and overall average number of mental health care visits per victimization were not derived.

Sources: Tjaden and Thoennes 2000; Bardwell Consulting, Ltd. (unpublished data) 2001; Max, Rice, Golding and Pinderhughes (unpublished data) 1999.

Table 6. Estimated Percentage of Victims and Number of Nonfatal Victimizations of Intimate Partner Rape, Physical Assault, and Stalking Against U.S. Adult Women, by Time Lost from Paid Work and Household Chores, 1995[a]

Victimization Type	Activity	Percent Victims	Number of Victimizations
Rape	Paid Work	21.5	69,279
	Household Chores	13.5	43,501
Physical assault	Paid Work	17.5	778,891
	Household Chores	10.3	458,433
Stalking	Paid Work	35.3	177,730
	Household Chores	17.5	88,110
TOTAL	**Paid Work**	**N/A**	**1,025,900**
	Household Chores	**N/A**	**590,044**

[a]Estimates are derived from the NVAWS based on the most recent intimate partner victimization since age 18.

NOTE: Victimization estimates of time lost from both paid work and household chores were derived separately for each victimization type. The total number of victimizations was subsequently derived by summing the respective estimates across victimization types. Consequently, the overall percentages of victims reporting time lost from paid work and household chores were not derived.

NOTE: See Appendix A for calculations of lost productivity and related values.

Sources: Tjaden and Thoennes (unpublished data) 1999;
Bardwell Consulting, Ltd. (unpublished data) 2001.

Intimate Partner Violence

Table 7. Estimated Lost Productivity Among U.S. Adult Female Victims of Nonfatal Intimate Partner Violence, by Victimization Type and by Time Lost from Paid Work and Household Chores, 1995[a]

| Victimization Type | Activity | Days Lost | | Lost Full-Time Job Equivalent[b] |
		Average	Total	
Rape	Paid Work	8.1	561,160	2,263
	Household Chores	13.5	587,264	N/A
Physical assault	Paid Work	7.2	5,608,015	22,613
	Household Chores	8.4	3,850,837	N/A
Stalking	Paid Work	10.1	1,795,073	7,238
	Household Chores	12.7	1,118,997	N/A
TOTAL	**Paid Work**	**N/A**	**7,964,248**	**32,114**
	Household Chores	**N/A**	**5,557,098**	**N/A**

[a]Estimates are derived from the NVAWS based on the most recent intimate partner victimization since age 18.

[b]The estimates of lost full-time job equivalents for paid work conservatively assume 248 work days per year.

NOTE: Victimization estimates of the average and total number of days lost from both paid work and household chores were derived separately for each victimization type. The overall total number of days lost was subsequently derived by summing the respective estimates across victimization types. Consequently, the overall average number of days lost from paid work and household chores were not derived.

NOTE: See Appendix A for illustrations of calculations of lost productivity and related values.

Sources: Tjaden and Thoennes (unpublished data) 1999;
Bardwell Consulting, Ltd. (unpublished data) 2001.

Costs of Intimate Partner Violence in the United States

Understanding the economic costs of intimate partner violence (IPV) can aid policy-makers in allocating resources more effectively and efficiently. This chapter provides the estimated annual costs of medical care, mental health care, lost productivity, and present value of lifetime earnings associated with IPV against U.S. adult women. The data presented reflect costs associated with IPV victimizations that occurred in 1995; these data are the most appropriate, reliable data currently available. It should be noted, however, that costs related to victimization in a given year are not always incurred in that year. For instance, mental health care visits related to IPV could continue for years after victimization. Therefore, estimated costs for victimization in a given year may underestimate the total costs of an incident of IPV victimization.

Calculating the Costs of Intimate Partner Violence

The economic costs of IPV are divided into two components—direct and indirect costs.

- **Direct costs** are the actual dollar expenditures related to IPV. They include spending for health care–related services such as emergency department (ED) visits; hospitalizations; outpatient clinic visits; services of physicians, dentists, physical therapists, and mental health professionals; ambulance transport; and paramedic assistance. To calculate the total costs of each medical and mental health care service, the unit cost of a particular service was multiplied by the number of times that service was used (Bardwell 2001).

- **Indirect costs** of IPV represent the value of lost productivity from both paid work and household chores for injured victims and the present value of lifetime earnings for victims of fatal IPV. Lost productivity was measured by the number of days victims were unable to perform paid work and/or household chores (including household chores and childcare for women not employed outside the home) because of illness, injury, or disability related to IPV victimization. The value of lost productivity was calculated using the mean daily values of work and household production, which are based on data from the U.S. Bureau of Labor Statistics (1996; 1999), Miller (1997), and the U.S. Bureau of the Census (1996). The present value of lifetime earnings was calculated by multiplying the number of IPV homicides for each age group by the average present value of the anticipated future earnings of women in those age groups. These calculations account for differential life expectancy by age group, labor force earning patterns and participation rates at successive ages, and imputed household production values for women in the labor force and women not in the labor force (Rice, Max, Golding and Pinderhughes 1997).

To yield more reliable estimates for service use and lost productivity, all most-recent IPV victimizations reported in the NVAWS—including those that occurred more than 12 months before the interview—were used to establish patterns of service use and lost productivity.

Data Sources Used to Calculate Costs of Intimate Partner Violence

As discussed previously, the National Violence Against Women Survey (NVAWS) and Uniform Crime Reports Supplementary Homicide Report were used to measure the incidence of fatal and nonfatal IPV, incidence of IPV-related health care service use among survivors, and lost productivity. Additionally, the following sources were used to calculate the health care costs of IPV:

- **Medical Expenditure Panel Survey (MEPS), 1996.** This survey by the Agency for Healthcare Research and Quality lists expenditures for medical care in the U.S. The MEPS is the main data source for unit costs of health care presented in this report. These unit costs were deflated to 1995 dollars using the appropriate health care components of the Consumer Price Index.

- **Medicare 5% Sample Beneficiary Standard Analytic Files.** This data source, which reflects physician/supplier claims, was used to calculate expenditures for ambulance and paramedic services, which are not available in MEPS.

Health Care Costs

In this report, service use estimates were restricted to services required as a result of the most recent victimizations by intimate partners, as derived from the NVAWS. In the NVAWS, only women who were injured as a result of IPV were asked about their use of medical care services. In contrast, all women who were victimized, regardless of injury, were asked about their use of mental health care services. Unit costs of medical and mental health care services for rape and physical assault victims were derived from the MEPS using medical and mental health visits related to injuries for women ages 18 and older. The unit costs of mental health care services for stalking victims were based on MEPS using mental health visits for women ages 18 and older who did not also sustain physical injuries.

Medical Care Costs

Medical care costs include ambulance transport and paramedic care; ED care; physician, physical therapy, and dental visits; inpatient hospitalizations; and outpatient clinic visits. Victims seeking medical care often received more than one service. We estimated the medical care costs of rape and physical assault separately. Rapes that involved physical assault were classified as rape only to avoid counting victimizations twice. No medical care costs were associated with stalking.

Rape. According to estimates from the NVAWS, 322,230 IPV rapes occur among women each year. Slightly more than one-third of these rapes (36.2%) result in physical injuries, 31.0% of which require medical care. In all, 36,161 IPV rapes result in women receiving medical care for injuries. Table 8 presents the number of times IPV rape victims use each medical care service, along with the unit costs of those services.

The mean medical care cost per IPV rape is about $516. The mean medical care cost per rape among victims who actually receive treatment is $2,084 per victimization. Not all victims who reported receiving medical care used all types of medical services. Therefore, the average cost of medical care for victims receiving treatment reflects variations in service use; it does not equal the total of each of the individual service costs per rape.

Nearly half of the medical care costs associated with IPV rape are paid by private or group insurance; victims pay more than one-quarter of the costs (Table 9).

Physical Assault. Based on NVAWS estimates, 4,450,807 IPV physical assaults occur against women annually; 41.5% of these assaults cause injuries. Medical care for injuries is required in 519,031 incidents (28.1% of those injured). Table 10 presents the number of times physical assault victims use medical care services and the unit costs of those services.

The mean medical care cost per incident of IPV physical assault is $548. The mean medical care cost per physical assault among victims who actually receive treatment is $2,665. Not all victims who reported receiving medical care used all types of medical services. Therefore, the average cost of medical care for victims receiving treatment reflects variations in service use; it does not equal the total of each of the individual service costs per physical assault.

As with IPV rape, private or group insurance pays for nearly half of medical care costs for IPV physical assaults; victims pay more than one-quarter of the costs (Table 9).

Mental Health Care Costs

All women in the NVAWS who reported IPV were asked if they used mental health care services. Because mental health care often requires multiple visits over a long period of time, the cost of these services is substantial.

Rape. According to NVAWS estimates, one-third (33.0%) of IPV rapes result in the victim's speaking with a psychologist, psychiatrist, or other mental health professional about the incident. On average, each incident requires 12.4 mental health care visits, for a total of 1.3 million mental health visits per year, at a mean cost of $78.86 per visit. The mean mental health care cost per incident of IPV rape is $323; the mean cost per IPV rape among victims who actually receive treatment is $978. Victims pay for more than one-third of mental health care services; private health insurers pay only slightly more than victims (Table 11).

Physical Assault. More than one-quarter (26.4%) of IPV physical assaults result in the victim's speaking with a psychologist, psychiatrist, or other mental health professional, according to NVAWS estimates. On average, each incident requires 12.9 visits, for a total of 15.2 million visits annually, at a mean cost of $78.86 per visit. The mean mental health care cost per incident of IPV physical assault, is $269; among victims who actually receive treatment, the mean cost per incident is $1,017. Victims pay for approximately one-third of the costs (Table 11).

Stalking. NVAWS estimates indicate than more than half a million women are stalked by intimate partners each year. Forty-three percent of these victims seek mental health care services, at an average of 9.6 visits per person. That's a total of nearly 2.1 million mental health care visits related to IPV stalking annually at a mean cost of $71.87 per visit. The mean mental health care cost per stalking incident by an intimate partner is $294; the mean cost per stalking incident among victims who actually receive treatment is $690. Private insurance pays for 34.7% of this mental health care; victims pay for 32.0% (Table 11).

Total Health Care Costs

The estimated total health care costs of IPV each year, including medical and mental health care services, is nearly $4.1 billion (Table 12). Of these costs, 89.7% are attributable to intimate partner physical assaults due to the large number of victimizations: 4,450,807 physical assaults compared with 322,230 rapes (6.7% of costs) and 503,485 stalking victimizations (3.7% of costs). The total medical and mental health care cost per victimization by an intimate partner was $838 per rape, $816 per physical assault, and $294 per stalking (Table 13).

Lost Productivity

Victims of IPV lose time from their regular activities due to injury and mental health issues. They may also be at greater risk for other health problems, such as chronic pain and sleep disturbances, which can interfere with or limit daily functioning (McCauley et al. 1995).

Rape. Among IPV rape victims, mean daily earnings lost are $69, and the mean daily value of household chores lost is $19.[1] According to NVAWS estimates, more than one-fifth (21.5%) of the women raped by an intimate partner report losing time from paid work, and 13.5% lose time from household chores (Table 14). Rape victims lose an estimated 1.1 million days of activity each year, which is equivalent to 3,872 person-years.

Physical assault. Among IPV physical assault victims, mean daily earnings lost are $93, and the mean daily value of household chores lost is $24. Approximately one in six (17.5%) victims report time lost from paid work, and 10.3% report lost time from household chores (Table 14). Victims of IPV physical assault lose an estimated 9.5 million days of activity each year; that equals 33,163 person-years of lost productivity.

Stalking. Among IPV stalking victims, mean daily earnings lost are $93, and the mean daily value of household chores lost is $24. More than one-third (35.3%) of stalking victims report time lost from paid work, according to NVAWS estimates; 17.5% report time lost from household chores (Table 14). Stalking victims lose an estimated 2.9 million days of productivity—or 10,304 person-years—annually.

Total Lost Productivity

As shown in Table 12, the estimated total value of days lost from employment and household chores is $858.6 million. The value of lost productivity from employment is $727.8 million, representing 84.8% of the total; the value of lost productivity from household chores is $130.8 million. More than 13.5 million total days are lost from job and housework productivity, which is equivalent to 47,339 person-years. Nearly three-quarters (71.6%) of lost productivity is due to physical assault; 22.6% of lost productivity is due to stalking.

Present Value of Lifetime Earnings

The present value of lifetime earnings (PVLE) measures the expected value of lost earnings that IPV homicide victims would have otherwise contributed to society had they been able to live out their full life expectancies. An estimated 1,252 women are killed by an intimate partner each year. The PVLE for these victims is an estimated $892.7 million—an average of more than $713,000 per fatality. (See Appendix B for PVLE by age group.)

---

[1]See Appendix A for calculations of lost productivity and related values as illustrated for rape estimates.

Intimate Partner Violence

Summary: Total Costs of Intimate Partner Violence

The costs of IPV against women exceed an estimated $5.8 billion (Table 12). These costs include nearly $4.1 billion in the direct costs of medical care and mental health care and nearly $1.8 billion in the indirect costs of lost productivity and PVLE. Statistically, the overall total cost estimate of $5.8 billion varies from more than $3.9 billion to more than $7.6 billion, as indicated by the 95% confidence interval for the total costs (Table 12).

The largest proportion of the costs is derived from physical assault victimizations because that type of IPV is the most prevalent (Figure 3). The largest component of IPV costs is health care, accounting for nearly $4.1 billion—more than two-thirds of the total costs (Figure 4).

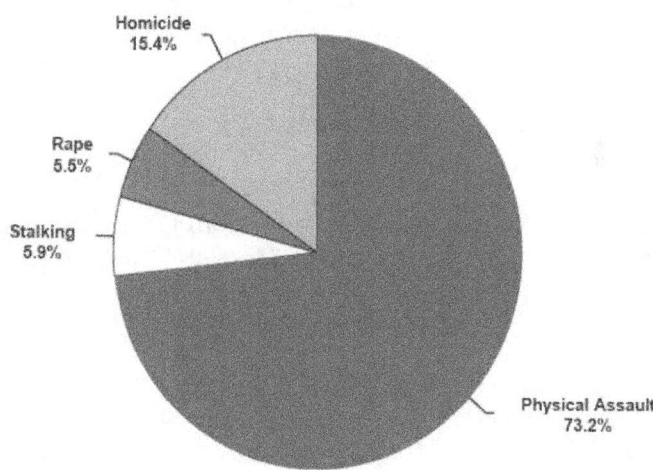

Figure 3.
Percentage of Costs of Intimate Partner Violence Against
U.S. Adult Women by Victimization Type, 1995

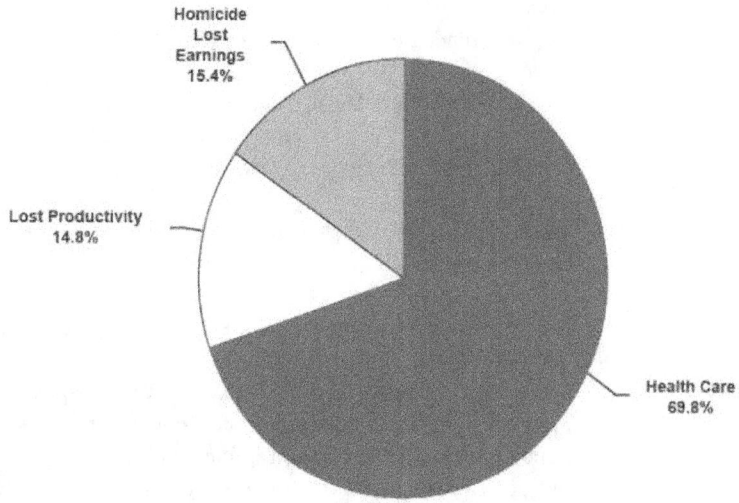

Figure 4.
Percentage of Costs of Intimate Partner Violence Against
U.S. Adult Women by Cost Type, 1995

Intimate Partner Violence

References

Bardwell Consulting, Ltd. *Final Report on Methodology for Computation of Confidence Intervals for Summary-Level Estimates in the Cost Study of Intimate Partner Violence Against Women;* July 2001. Final report for task order 0621-15, funded by the Centers for Disease Control and Prevention.

Bardwell Consulting, Ltd. Unpublished data for task order 0621-15, funded by the Centers for Disease Control and Prevention; 2001.

Max W, Rice DP, Golding J, Pinderhughes H. *Cost of Intimate Partner Violence Against Women in the United States, 1995;* 1999. Report for contract 282-92-0048, funded by the Office of the Assistant Secretary for Planning and Evaluation and the Centers for Disease Control and Prevention, U.S. Department of Health and Human Services.

McCauley J, Kern DK, Kolodner K, Dill L, Schroeder AF, DeChant HK, et al. The "battering syndrome": prevalence and clinical characteristics of domestic violence in primary care internal medicine practices. *Annals of Internal Medicine* 1995;123:737–46.

Miller T. Unpublished data on the value of household production. Landover (MD): National Public Services Research Institute; 1997.

Office of Statistics and Programming, National Center for Injury Prevention and Control, Centers for Disease Control and Prevention. Collapsed total cost summary estimates of intimate partner violence. Unpublished data; 2002.

Research Triangle Institute International. *Methodology Used to Produce Select Unit Cost Estimates, Variance Estimates, and Confidence Intervals,* 2001. Report for task order 0621-15, funded by the Centers for Disease Control and Prevention.

Rice D, Max W, Golding J, Pinderhughes H. *The Cost of Domestic Violence to the Health Care System. Final Report.* Report prepared for the Office of the Assistant Secretary for Planning and Evaluation, U.S. Department of Health and Human Services; 1997.

Tjaden P, Thoennes N. *Prevalence, Incidence, and Consequences of Intimate Partner Violence Against Women: Findings from the National Violence Against Women Survey;* 1999. Unpublished report for grant 93-IJ-CX-0012, funded by the U.S. Department of Justice, National Institute of Justice; and the Centers for Disease Control and Prevention.

Tjaden P, Thoennes N. *Extent, Nature, and Consequences of Intimate Partner Violence: Findings from the National Violence Against Women Survey, Research Report,* 2000. Report for grant 93-IJ-CX-0012, funded by the U.S. Department of Justice, National Institute of Justice; and the Centers for Disease Control and Prevention. NCJ 181867.

U.S. Bureau of the Census, U.S. Department of Commerce. *Money Income in the United States: 1995.* Current Population Reports, P60-193. Washington (DC): U.S. Government Printing Office; 1996.

U.S. Bureau of Labor Statistics, U.S. Department of Labor. *Employment and Earnings. January 1994.* Washington (DC): U.S. Government Printing Office; 1996.

U.S. Bureau of Labor Statistics, U.S. Department of Labor. *National Compensation Survey: Occupational Wages in the United States, 1997.* Washington (DC): U.S. Government Printing Office; 1999.

Table 8. Estimated Medical Care Service Use and Unit Costs for Nonfatal Intimate Partner Rape Against U.S. Adult Women, 1995

| | | | | | Cost Per Rape | |
Type of Medical Service	No. of Rapes Requiring Medical Care	Average No. of Uses Per Rape	Total Uses	Unit Cost for Service	All Rapes[a]	Rapes Requiring Medical Care
ED visits	14,766	1.9	28,055	$ 346.73	$ 30.19	$ 658.79
Outpatient visits	8,865	1.6	14,184	347.59	15.30	556.14
Hospital overnights	12,550	3.9	48,945	2,519.90[b]	382.76	9,827.61
Physician visits	21,407	5.2	111,316	112.21	38.76	583.49
Dental visits	6,654	2.3	15,304	308.90[b]	14.67	710.46
Ambulance/paramedic services	7,377	1.3	9,590	121.13	3.60	157.46
Physical therapy visits	8,100	13.4	108,540	89.74	30.23	1,202.52

[a]To determine the cost per rape across all rapes, the total cost associated with each medical care service is divided by the estimated total number of intimate partner rapes (322,230), whether or not the victim was injured.

[b]The unit cost estimates of hospital overnights and dental visits are unstable and are used only as part of intermediate calculations.

Sources: Max, Rice, Golding and Pinderhughes 1999; Research Triangle Institute International 2001; Bardwell Consulting, Ltd. (unpublished data) 2001; Tjaden and Thoennes 2000.

Table 9. Distribution of Primary Source of Payment for Medical Care Resulting from Nonfatal Intimate Partner Rape and Physical Assault Against U.S. Adult Women, 1995

Payer	Rape Victims (Percent Paid)	Physical Assault Victims (Percent Paid)
Medicare	N/A[a]	3.0
Medicaid	12.5	11.0
Private or group insurance	45.8	48.3
Out of pocket	29.2	28.6
Free or low-income clinics	2.1	1.8
Other public sources	10.4	6.1
Some other source	N/A[a]	1.2
TOTAL	**100.0**	**100.0**

[a]Among the reported rape cases in the NVAWS that resulted in injury and medical care, no payments were made by Medicare or "some other source." However, analysts assume that among the total rapes resulting in injury and treatment in the U.S., these payment categories are not actually 0%. Therefore, the estimates are considered unavailable. To determine the percentage distribution of the remaining payment categories, the categories with unavailable estimates were ignored.

Source: Tjaden and Thoennes (unpublished data) 1999.

Intimate Partner Violence

Table 10. Estimated Medical Care Service Use and Unit Costs for Nonfatal Intimate Partner Physical Assault Against U.S. Adult Women, 1995

Type of Service	No. of Physical Assaults Requiring Medical Care	Average No. of Uses Per Assault	No. of Uses	Unit Cost for Service	Cost Per Physical Assault	
					All Physical Assaults[a]	Physical Assaults Requiring Medical Care
ED visits	241,103	1.9	458,096	$ 346.73	$ 35.69	$ 658.79
Outpatient visits	98,726	3.1	306,051	347.59	23.90	1,077.53
Hospital overnights	132,994	5.7	758,066	2,519.90	429.19	14,363.43
Physician visits	268,858	3.2	860,346	112.21	21.69	359.07
Dental visits	49,308	4.4	216,955	308.90	15.06	1,359.16
Ambulance/paramedic services	77,336	1.1	85,070	121.13	2.32	133.24
Physical therapy visits	46,194	21.1	974,693	89.74	19.65	1,893.51

[a]To determine the cost per physical assault across all physical assaults, the total cost associated with each medical care service is divided by the estimated total number of intimate partner physical assault victimizations (4,450,807), whether or not the victim was injured.

Sources: Max, Rice, Golding and Pinderhughes 1999; Research Triangle Institute International 2001; Bardwell Consulting, Ltd. (unpublished data) 2001; Tjaden and Thoennes 2000.

Table 11. Distribution of Primary Source of Payment for Mental Health Care Resulting from Intimate Partner Rape, Physical Assault, and Stalking Against U.S. Adult Women, 1995

Payer	Rape Victims (Percent Paid)	Physical Assault Victims (Percent Paid)	Stalking Victims (Percent Paid)
Medicare	2.1	1.9	2.8
Medicaid	10.5	6.9	11.1
Private or group insurance	37.1	43.1	34.7
Out-of-Pocket	33.6	32.0	32.0
Free or low-income clinics	10.5	11.6	15.3
Some other source	2.8	1.6	N/A[a]
Other public sources	3.5	2.9	4.2
TOTAL[b]	**100.0**	**100.0**	**100.0**

[a]Among the victimizations of stalking in the NVAWS that resulted in mental health care, no payments were made by "some other source." However, analysts assume that among the total stalking victimizations resulting in mental health care in the U.S., this payment category is not actually 0%. Therefore, the estimate is considered unavailable. To determine the percentage distribution of the remaining payment categories, the "some other source" category estimate was ignored.

[b]Columns may not sum due to rounding.

Source: Tjaden and Thoennes (unpublished data) 1999.

Intimate Partner Violence

Table 12. Estimated Total Costs of intimate Partner Violence Against U.S. Adult Women, 1995

Type of Cost	Estimated Total Cost (in Thousands)	Total Cost 95% Confidence interval (in Thousands)	
		Lower Limit	Upper Limit
Health care[a]	$ 4,050,211	$ 2,207,491	$ 5,892,931
Lost productivity	$ 858,618	$ 596,058	$ 1,121,178
Paid work	$ 727,831	$ 470,435	$ 985,227
Household chores[b]	$ 130,787	$ 78,969	$ 182,605
Present value of lifetime earnings	$ 892,733	$ 839,723	$ 945,743
TOTAL COSTS (Direct + Indirect)	$ 5,801,561	$ 3,939,475	$ 7,633,648

[a]Health care costs include mental health and medical care costs. In turn, medical care costs include outpatient clinic visits; emergency department visits; ambulance transport or paramedic care; physician, physical therapy, and dental visits; and inpatient hospitalization.

[b]The productivity value for household chores was discounted for victims who also worked at a job for pay. Due to the uncertain labor force status of victims who reported only lost productivity from household chores, one cannot assume that these victims were necessarily out of the labor force. Consequently, the value assigned to all lost productivity from household chores was discounted.

NOTE: The Estimated Total Cost column does not sum to Total Costs due to rounding.

Sources: CDC, NCIPC, Office of Statistics and Programming (unpublished data) 2002; Bardwell 2001; Bardwell Consulting, Ltd. (unpublished data) 2001; Max, Rice, Golding and Pinderhughes 1999; Research Triangle Institute International 2001.

Table 13. Estimated Average Health Care Costs per Nonfatal Intimate Partner Rape, Physical Assault, and Stalking Victimization Against U.S. Adult Women, 1995

Health Care Costs	Rape[a]	Physical Assault[a]	Stalking[a]
Medical Care, Total[b]	$ 515.51	$ 547.50	N/A
ED visits	30.19	35.69	N/A
Outpatient visits	15.30	23.90	N/A
Hospital overnights	382.76	429.19	N/A
Physician visits	38.76	21.69	N/A
Dental visits	14.67	15.06	N/A
Ambulance/paramedic services	3.60	2.32	N/A
Physical therapy visits	30.23	19.65	N/A
Mental Health Care, Total	$ 322.70	$ 268.57	$ 293.92
TOTAL	$ 838.21	$ 816.07	$ 293.92

[a]Estimates are based on 322,230 rapes, 4,450,807 physical assaults, and 503,485 stalking incidents.
[b]No medical care costs are associated with stalking.

Sources: Max, Rice, Golding and Pinderhughes 1999; Research Triangle Institute International 2001; Tjaden and Thoennes 2000.

Table 14. Estimated Lost Productivity Due to Intimate Partner Rape, Physical Assault, and Stalking Against U.S. Adult Women by Victimization Type, 1995

Victimization Type	Paid Work	Household Chores	Total
Rape			
Percentage of victims reporting days lost	21.5	13.5	N/A
Mean number of days lost per rape[a]	8.1	13.5	N/A
Total Days Lost[a]	**561,000**	**587,000**	**1,148,000**
Physical Assault			
Percentage of victims reporting days lost	17.5	10.3	N/A
Mean number of days lost per physical assault[a]	7.2	8.4	N/A
Total Days Lost[a]	**5,608,000**	**3,851,000**	**9,459,000**
Stalking			
Percentage of victims reporting days lost	35.3	17.5	N/A
Mean number of days lost per stalking[a]	10.1	12.7	N/A
Total Days Lost[a]	**1,795,000**	**1,119,000**	**2,914,000**

[a]Among victims who returned to the reported activity.

NOTE: The estimated total number of victimizations for rape is 322,230; for physical assault, 4,450,807; and for stalking, 503,485.

NOTE: For each type of victimization, the percentage of victims reporting days lost and the mean number of days lost per victimization differ between those victims who lost time from paid work and those victims who lost time from household chores. Consequently, the number of days lost from paid work and household chores must be determined separately, then totaled to obtain the total of days lost for each vicitimization type. As a result, the total or overall percentage of victims reporting days lost and the overall mean number of days lost per vicitimization were not calculated.

NOTE: See Appendix A for illustrations of calculations of lost productivity and related values.

Sources: Max, Rice, Golding and Pinderhughes 1999; Research Triangle Institute International 2001; Tjaden and Thoennes (unpublished data) 1999.

Discussion

This report presents estimates of the incidence, prevalence, and costs of intimate partner violence against U.S. women ages 18 and older. In addition to data about IPV fatalities obtained from existing FBI sources, it uses data from the first large-scale survey to collect information about injuries IPV victims sustained, the medical and mental health care services victims used, and the time victims lost from paid work and household chores. The report reflects the most appropriate, reliable data currently available about the costs associated with IPV. Standard public health methods were applied to recent data on IPV-related injuries to estimate their incidence, estimate resulting health care costs and lost productivity, and to review strategies for reducing the incidence of IPV.

As reported in previous chapters, nearly 5.3 million intimate partner victimizations occur each year among U.S. women ages 18 and older, and nearly 1,300 women lose their lives as a result of IPV. Based on these estimates, such violence costs our nation more than an estimated $5.8 billion dollars annually—nearly $4.1 billion for medical and mental health care, $0.9 billion in lost productivity, and $0.9 billion in homicide lost earnings. These figures are believed to underestimate the problem of IPV for many reasons, and additional efforts are needed to better determine the costs of IPV against women in the U.S.

Using the Cost Figures in this Report

The cost estimates presented in this report can be used to—

- Calculate the economic cost savings from reducing a given number of injuries resulting from IPV;

- Demonstrate the economic magnitude of IPV in the U.S.;

- Evaluate the impact of IPV on a specific sub-sector of the economy, such as consumption of medical resources or effects on employers.

However, because of some limitations in the data—the discussion of which follows—these estimates are not comprehensive. Therefore, the estimates in this report should not be used in direct comparisons with the costs of reducing IPV, namely to produce benefit-cost ratios in analyses of interventions to prevent IPV.

Data Limitations

The cost estimates presented in this report have several limitations, the most obvious of which is the fact that 1995 incidence data were used to generate annual estimates. CDC recognizes that direct costs, value of lost productivity, and present value of lifetime earnings resulting from IPV today may differ from that of IPV that occurred in 1995. However, this report reflects the most appropriate, reliable data available to date about the costs associated with IPV. Other limitations involve the exclusion of certain costs potentially associated with IPV and the use of average rather than actual medical care costs.

Excluded Costs

Several cost components were excluded from this report because data were unavailable or insufficient. Perhaps the largest omission is criminal justice costs. NVAWS data indicate that an estimated 1.5 million intimate partner rape, physical assault, or stalking victimizations result in police reports each year; nearly 79,000 of these victimizations result in a jail or prison sentence. While IPV-related criminal justice service use is significant, current data about unit costs do not allow for reliable, nationally representative cost estimates associated with these services.

Some medical care costs, including home care visits, treatment for sexually transmitted diseases (STDs), and terminated pregnancies were excluded because there were too few victimizations resulting in these outcomes reported in the NVAWS to generate reliable cost estimates. Also excluded were cost components for which either no data were available or only incidence data were available: social services such as women's shelters and counseling clinics; shelter, moral support, and financial assistance from IPV victims' friends and family; medical or mental health costs of treating children who witness IPV; foster care for children as a result of IPV; and the value of time lost from volunteer work, school, and social and recreational activities.

Although the mental health care costs associated with IPV were calculated, it was not possible to estimate the intangible costs of pain and suffering associated with IPV that did not result in a mental health care visit, or that did not result in a visit where IPV was identified as associated with the suffering. Because costs of this type may be quite high, this report should be viewed as presenting very conservative estimates, or as the lower limit of the costs related to IPV.

Because the NVAWS reports on the survivors of IPV, data about victims' use of medical and mental health services were collected only for victims of nonfatal IPV. No data were collected about the health care costs associated with treating victims who ultimately die as a result of IPV.

Limitations of the
Medical Care Data

Health care service use resulting from IPV is not always readily reported. Therefore, the health care costs in this report are underestimates and should be viewed as lower limits of the magnitude of the problem.

Evidence has shown that victims of IPV manifest a wide range of physical symptoms that are not directly related to abuse. These can include headaches, reproductive health problems, chronic pain, digestive problems, and sleep disturbances (McCauley et al. 1995). To the extent that medical care service use associated with indirect physical symptoms of IPV was not reported by victims, related costs are excluded from the health care estimates in this report.

Limitations of the
Mental Health Care Data

Data about mental health–related costs of IPV are limited for several reasons. First, incidence estimates derived from the NVAWS are based on the response to a question about whether or not the victim spoke to a mental health professional. As no definition of mental health professional was given, this question was subject to the interpretation of the respondent. Furthermore, mental health professionals are not the only individuals from whom victims may seek mental health care.

Second, respondents were asked only about mental health care providers with whom they discussed their experience of IPV victimization. Some women may have sought care for mental health problems but not identified that it was related to past experiences of IPV.

Finally, the cost of unmet mental health needs is not estimated. This is a critical gap in IPV research because the violence itself may limit women's use of needed services. That is, men who physically abuse their partners are also likely to control and coerce them (Wilson, Johnson and Daly 1995), including restricting their access to mental health care (Walker 1984).

Underestimate of a
Particular Type of Victimization

Although some incidents involved more than one type of victimization (e.g., a woman whose former husband stalks and then rapes her), the NVAWS counted each incident only once and classified it according to the severity of abuse. Rape was considered more severe than physical assault, and physical assault more severe than stalking. Women who sustained injuries during incidents involving more than one type of victimization were asked to report services used as a result of these injuries for the most severe type of victimization involved in these incidents. They were asked not to report service use for the same injuries when asked about the less severe type(s) of victimization involved in the particular incident. These procedures prevented double-counting of both service use and associated costs resulting from these incidents. However, these procedures likely resulted in an underestimate of health care costs resulting from physical assault, because some costs are included under rape. Likewise, some stalking costs are likely included under physical assault and rape.

Conservative Cost Estimation

The cost estimates of IPV in this report are generally conservative for several reasons. First, the NVAWS estimates of IPV victimization among women are lower than estimates in other studies. Second, the estimates presented in this report are based on services that victims of IPV reported using. Some NVAWS respondents may not have reported IPV due to embarrassment or shame. Consequently, any services used as a result of these victimizations also went unreported.

Finally, the estimate of present value of lifetime earnings relies on criminal homicide data that include the relationship between victim and perpetrator and the victim's age. The relationship between victim and perpetrator was not known for all homicide cases, which likely results in an undercounting of IPV homicides. Additionally, about 1% of homicide cases determined to be the result of IPV did not report victim's age. The present value of lifetime earnings could not be calculated for those cases, thus resulting in a conservative estimate.

A Need for More Data

This report is an important step in understanding the current knowledge about intimate partner violence in the U.S. However, it highlights a need for more data to fully appreciate the economic and human costs of this problem. Obtaining these data will involve creating standard definitions of IPV, expanding quantitative data collection efforts, and employing methods to gather qualitative data.

Standardizing the Definition of Intimate Partner Violence

Definitions of intimate partner violence vary among agencies collecting data. For example, some definitions include same sex partners, and some do not. Some consider IPV among both current and former intimate partners, some do not. Because of these variations, survey data also vary, making it difficult to firmly state the magnitude of IPV.

To address problems posed by varying definitions, CDC recently facilitated a national process to develop standard definitions of IPV (Saltzman et al. 1999). At the same time, CDC funded several states to develop IPV surveillance systems that use these definitions to gather data from the health care, social service, and criminal justice systems. This project serves as a pilot test of the IPV definitions and the feasibility of developing statewide public health surveillance to estimate the magnitude of the problem.

Improving Quantitative Data

The information about service use provided in this report includes medical and mental health care obtained from the traditional medical care system. Many survivors of IPV do not seek out these health care providers, especially for mental health care. Instead, they may go to support groups and rape crisis centers or contact crisis hotlines. Researchers should find ways to gather data from such service providers. Additionally, many women experience repeated IPV victimizations, yet little is known about the cumulative effects of such repeat abuse on service use.

One area for which costs of IPV may be substantial is criminal justice services. The NVAWS asked survivors about their involvement with the criminal justice system, but inadequate unit cost data exist to allow for generating unbiased estimates of the costs of those services. In fact, only one county at the time of the survey had unit cost data. Nationally representative data about the costs of individual criminal justice services—police reports, arrests and detainment, legal and judicial services, incarceration, probation—are needed.

While health system data about IPV, primarily derived from hospital discharge and emergency department records, have improved in recent years, future efforts will allow for even better data collection. The clinical modification of ICD-10 (ICD-10 CM) will provide information about abuse, neglect, abandonment, and the perpetrator's relationship to the victim. This will enable better IPV data collection from health sources.

Collecting Qualitative Data

Perhaps more compelling than the economic costs are data about the human costs. But how do you quantify pain, suffering, and decreased quality of life associated with intimate partner violence, both on survivors and on children exposed to such violence? Data are needed to assess the long-term, psychosocial effects of IPV and to demonstrate more clearly the social burden of this problem. Researchers should explore methods for collecting data about indirect or intangible costs of IPV, such as using in-depth interviews with survivors and service providers.

Intimate Partner Violence

A Need for Primary Prevention of Intimate Partner Violence

To reduce both the economic and human costs of intimate partner violence against women, we must focus on primary prevention—finding ways to stop such violence before it ever occurs—rather than only treating victims and rehabilitating perpetrators. To that end, CDC has identified several priorities to address IPV prevention. These priorities, set forth in CDC's *Injury Research Agenda*, represent the research issues that warrant the greatest attention and extramural and intramural research from CDC for the next three to five years. (The agenda can be viewed online at: www.cdc.gov/ncipc/pub-res/research_agenda/agenda.htm.)

One key area of CDC's IPV research is social norms. Social norms—what a community views as acceptable behaviors for its citizens—can profoundly affect efforts to prevent public health problems. In October 2000, CDC began exploring how social norms affect intimate partner violence. Findings are guiding development of a campaign to change social norms that accept or promote IPV against women. The campaign will target boys in sixth through eighth grades, a population in which strong social norms are developing quickly and in which we can effect lasting changes. It will focus on the characteristics of healthy relationships, in which violence is unacceptable.

CDC is also working to find ways to intervene with individuals, families, and communities in ways that stop violence before it happens. Its research agenda calls for developing programs and policies that provide counseling for batterers and prevent dating violence as means of intervening with perpetrators and potential perpetrators. The agenda also sets a priority to better understand how violent behavior toward intimate partners develops, so that researchers can implement strategies to reduce factors that increase the risk of IPV perpetration.

Other areas of research about preventing intimate partner violence include developing and evaluating training programs about IPV detection and prevention for health professionals, evaluating the health consequences of IPV across the life span, developing and evaluating surveillance methods to better collect data about incidence and prevalence of IPV, and disseminating information about IPV prevention strategies that work.

Conclusion

With an estimated economic cost of $5.8 billion, and the untold intangible costs, intimate partner violence against women is a substantial public health problem that must be addressed. Significant resources for research are needed to better understand the magnitude, causes. and risk factors of IPV and to develop and disseminate effective primary prevention strategies. Until we reduce the incidence of IPV in the United States, we will not reduce the economic and social burden of this problem.

References

McCauley J, Kern DK, Kolodner K, Dill L, Schroeder AF, DeChant HK, et al. The "battering syndrome": prevalence and clinical characteristics of domestic violence in primary care internal medicine practices. *Annals of Internal Medicine* 1995;123:737–46.

Saltzman LE, Fanslow JL, McMahon PM, Shelley GA. *Intimate Partner Violence Surveillance: Uniform definitions and recommended data elements, Version 1.0*. Atlanta: Centers for Disease Control and Prevention, National Center for Injury Prevention and Control; 1999.

Walker LE. *The Battered Woman Syndrome*. New York: Springer; 1984.

Wilson M, Johnson F, Daly M. Lethal and nonlethal violence against wives. *Canadian Journal of Criminology* 1995;37:331–61.

Intimate Partner Violence

Appendix A

Calculating Lost Productivity and Related Values

Total Days Lost from Paid Work and Household Chores

To determine the total days lost from paid work and household chores for each victimization type, we first determined the total number of victimizations that resulted in days lost from each of those activities:

Percent victimizations resulting in days lost X
Total number of victimizations =
Total number of victimizations resulting in days lost.

For example, to determine the number IPV rape victimizations that resulted in lost paid work:

21.5% of rapes resulting in days lost from paid work X
322,230 total rape victimizations =
69,279 rapes resulting in days lost from paid work.

Next, multiply the number of victimizations resulting in lost days of a given activity by the mean number of days lost from that activity per victimization. For example, to determine the total number of paid work days lost for rape victimizations:

69,279 rapes resulting in lost paid work days X
8.1 mean number of days lost from paid work per rape =
Approximately 561,000 total days lost
from paid work due to rape victimization.

Person-Years Lost from Paid Work
and Household Chores

Total time lost may also be expressed in person-years lost. For paid work, these calculations assumed 248 work days per year; for household chores, 365 days per year. To calculate person-years:

Total number of days lost for a given activity for a given victimization type /
Number of productivity days per year =
Total person-years lost for that victimization type.

For example, to calculate person-years of household chores lost for rape victimizations:

561,000 total days lost / 365 days of household chores =
2,262 person-years lost.

NOTE: Total person-years presented here may be slightly different than those presented elsewhere in this report; rounded figures are used here, but unrounded estimates were used elsewhere.

Mean Daily Values and Total Value of
Lost Productivity

To estimate the total value of lost productivity for each victimization type, we need to first estimate the respective mean daily value of earnings from work. Mean daily values of earnings are based on the mean age of women at the time of victimization. For rape, the mean age at the time of victimization is 24.5 years; for physical assault, 27.5 years; and for stalking, 26.5 years (Max, Rice, Golding and Pinderhughes 1999). For each victimization type, the mean daily value of earnings is, in turn, based on the respective mean annual earnings for women of the mean victimization age group (U.S. Bureau of Census 1996; U.S. Bureau of Labor Statistics 1996).

To calculate the mean daily value of earnings for each victimization type:

Mean annual earnings of the mean victimization age group /
Number of paid work days per year =
Mean daily value of earnings.

For example, to calculate the mean daily value of earnings for rape victims:

$17,058 (mean annual earnings for mean victimization age) /
248 paid work days per year =
$68.78 daily value.

To calculate the total value of lost days from paid work:

Mean daily value of earnings X total days of earnings lost =
Total value of lost days.

For example, for rape victimizations:

$68.78 X 561,000 total days of earnings lost due to rape =
Approximately $38,600,000.

Follow the same calculations to determine the total value of days lost from household chores.

References

Max W, Rice DP, Golding J, Pinderhughes H. *Cost of Intimate Partner Violence Against Women in the United States, 1995*; 1999. Report for contract 282-92-0048, funded by the Office of the Assistant Secretary for Planning and Evaluation and the Centers for Disease Control and Prevention, U.S. Department of Health and Human Services.

U.S. Bureau of the Census, U.S. Department of Commerce. *Money Income in the United States: 1995*. Current Population Reports, P60-193. Washington (DC): U.S. Government Printing Office; 1996.

U.S. Bureau of Labor Statistics, U.S. Department of Labor. *Employment and Earnings. January 1994*. Washington (DC): U.S. Government Printing Office; 1996.

Intimate Partner Violence

Appendix B

Calculating Age Group–Specific Present Value of Lifetime Earnings Estimates

Present Value of Lifetime Earnings (PVLE) Among Adult Female Victims of
Intimate Partner Homicide by Age Group, U.S., 1995

Age Group	No. of Homicides	Mean PVLE	Total PVLE
18–19	50	$ 938,545	$ 46,927,268
20–24	176	958,434	168,684,384
25–29	182	924,842	168,321,244
30–34	217	852,312	184,951,704
35–39	207	754,284	156,136,788
40–44	148	637,849	94,401,652
45–49	73	509,876	37,220,948
50–54	58	380,019	22,041,102
55–59	26	257,641	6,698,666
60–64	23	156,178	3,592,094
65–69	24	86,713	2,081,112
70–74	22	45,029	990,638
75–79	25	21,336	533,400
80–84	16	8,682	138,912
85 and older	5	2,557	12,785
OVERALL TOTAL	1,252	N/A	$ 892,732,697

NOTE: The mean PVLE for each age group was multiplied by the number of intimate partner homicides in that age group to arrive at the total PVLE for that group. Then, all age group–specific PVLEs were added to arrive at the overall total PVLE.